IGOR G.

Boxing Home Workouts For Beginners

Discover Simple Yet Powerful Workouts To Keep You Fit and Motivated

First edition

This book was professionally typeset on Reedsy.
Find out more at reedsy.com

"Don't ever quit on yourself, no matter how hard it gets. Give it 100% in boxing, and it'll translate to 100% in other areas of your life!"

– Anonymous Boxing Coach

Contents

1

Introduction

Did you know that boxing not only teaches self-defense but also builds unparalleled fitness levels? Welcome to BOXING HOME WORKOUTS FOR BEGINNERS! My name is Igor Ganapolsky, and I am an amateur boxer. I am very enthusiastic to be writing this book! Firstly, now I'll have a guide for my own boxing workouts, and share it with friends and family who do these types of workouts at home. Second, I can share this simple regimen with other beginners who want to get fit, because I was a beginner boxer not long ago too. Third, boxing has given me so much joy in my life that it's an addiction. It has made me as fit and slim as I've ever been, and I am now in my 40s!

How I got into boxing: I started my youth training and competed in other martial arts (Tae Kwon Do and Tang Soo Do). While good for kicking, these arts didn't address the need for punching with power and skill. As a result, my self-defense ability with hands failed me and I wasn't conditioned to get into a fist fight. In my adult life I played sports (basketball, running) and weight-lifted in the gym. While these sports made my endurance and cardio better and built muscle, I still couldn't go all out in a real self-defense scenario involving fists. When I turned 40 I began training in mixed martial arts (Jiu Jitsu, Krav Maga, Kickboxing, Combatives, Wing Chun, Systema). These are all great arts, but still my endurance and confidence and using my fists in a real fight were lacking.

A friend then recommended I try boxing, primarily to improve my footwork. I joined a nearby boxing studio and fell in love with the sport from day 1! The workouts were an hour and a half long, non-stop endurance & conditioning, and my punching skill and power grew with each training session. I was attending four classes per week and supplemented these training sessions at home with a self-made gym in my garage. Additionally, I ran three miles four times per week, which gave my cardio a tremendous boost. As time went on, I joined the competition team at the studio and began sparring regularly in the ring, with the intent to compete in the masters division one day.

Beginners want a solid foundation on boxing techniques and workouts without feeling overwhelmed. Boxing is an appealing and accessible fitness regimen. If you are a beginner, then I want to empower you with the knowledge and tools needed to start boxing. You probably want quick progression and fitness goals. And you likely desire a systematic guide that will help you see tangible results and improvement in your boxing skills and overall fitness. I aim to support you in reaching these ideals with this book.

Who This Book Is For

This book is for anybody at any age who wants to get more fit, and is inspired by boxing routines they have seen. Anybody who has a healthy enough body to throw light punches, jog at their own pace, jump rope at their own speed, and do a few push-ups and sit-ups. Most importantly, anybody who values getting fit through a functional fighting art, which disciplines the mind and makes the body more resilient in this tough world.

Also, if you are an aspiring athlete who wants to compete in boxing one day or who wants to spar in the ring, you will greatly benefit from doing these routines regularly.

2

What To Expect, Pre-Workout Planning

What To Expect

Safety and Injury Prevention: Knowing how to train safely and minimize the risk of injury is paramount for new enthusiasts. It is paramount that you listen to your body and progress incrementally rather than push it to the point of injury. If you follow the laid out workouts approximately four days per week, at your own pace, you'll see a vast improvement in the following:

Cardiovascular Health Improvement: Boxing is a high-intensity workout that keeps your heart rate elevated. This helps in improving cardiovascular health. For beginners, starting with shorter rounds and gradually increasing time and intensity can make it more accessible.

Weight Loss and Muscle Tone: Boxing burns a significant number of calories, helping in weight loss. It also targets various muscle groups, helping in toning the body. A beginner may start with basic punches and combinations and slowly add more complex moves as they progress.

Enhanced Hand-Eye Coordination: Boxing requires precise timing and coordination. Practicing with a speed bag or focusing mitts can significantly enhance hand-eye coordination. Even beginners will notice this improvement with consistent practice.

Stress Reduction: Boxing can be an excellent outlet for stress, allowing one to channel energy into a physical activity. Creating a routine and sticking to it can help newcomers find a healthy way to deal with daily stress.

Improvement in Body Strength: Boxing is not just about punches; it's about using the whole body. Core strength is often enhanced through the movements in boxing. Beginners can incorporate exercises like planks and core rotations into their boxing workout to build strength gradually.

Increased Self-Confidence: Learning a new skill like boxing can boost self-esteem and confidence. Setting realistic goals and achieving them can be very satisfying for a beginner.

Flexibility and Agility Enhancement: Boxing requires quick movements, footwork, and flexibility. Incorporating stretching and agility drills into the workout can help improve these areas over time.

Pre-Workout Planning

Equipment: The equipment you'll need to get the most out of your boxing workouts is as follows:

- Comfortable workout clothing that you can stretch, run, and sweat in.
- Good running shoes in which you can run and walk several miles.
- Boxing gloves - 10 oz gloves if you weigh less than 150 lbs, and 16 oz gloves if you weigh more than 150 lbs.
- Boxing hand wraps (for wearing inside gloves). There are many YouTube videos which will show you how to wrap your hands.
- Heavy bag (approximately half your body weight).
- Resistance Stretch Band. Start with a 2-15 lbs band, and get more resistance as you get stronger.
- Jump rope. The right length for a jump rope is about 10-12 inches above your head. Another way to select a jump rope is one that reaches up to your armpits when standing on the middle of it.
- Foam roller.

Space for Practice: You'll need a park, pedestrian street or a stadium where you can jump rope and run on. A garage to hang a heavy bag from a beam or put a standing heavy bag on the floor. If you don't have a garage, then you can use a backyard or a large room. A floor where you can do your stretching and foam rolling.

Time for Practice: Set aside at least one hour for your workout routine, at least three days per week. I do my workouts at different times throughout the day: running in the morning, boxing at the studio in the evening, push-ups and stretching throughout the day at home.

3

Warmups On The Jump Rope

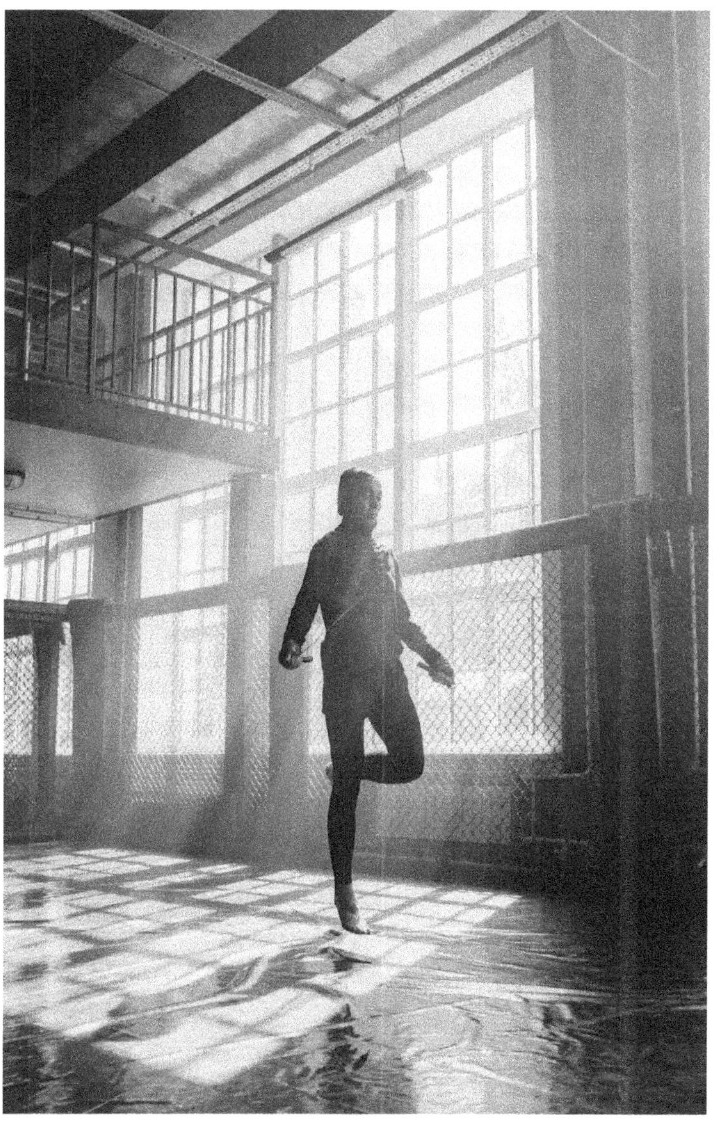

Jump Rope Warmups to Get Light on Your Feet

At the boxing studio, we always start our practice with nine minutes of jump rope (three rounds of 3 minutes, with 30 second breaks in between). I have grown to appreciate the jump rope and what it offers for boxers: getting light on your feet, breaking a sweat, building cardio. I recommend that you start your boxing workouts with at least three minutes of jump rope, and then build up to six and nine minutes. Here's a step-by-step guide to some beginner-friendly jump rope exercises suitable for your workouts:

1. Basic Jump Rope (Single Bounce)
   Hold the jump rope handles with your hands slightly above waist level.
   Keep your elbows close to your body.
   Use your wrists to turn the rope, not your arms.
   Jump off the ground just high enough to clear the rope.
   Land softly on the balls of your feet.
   Keep a steady rhythm and try to do this continuously.

2. Alternate Foot Step (Running in Place)
   Just like the basic jump, but alternate lifting your knees.
   You'll essentially be running in place as you jump the rope.
   Keep your knees high and your jumps small to maintain a fast pace.

3. Side-to-Side Jump
   Perform the basic jump rope technique.
   As you jump, move your feet slightly to the left and then slightly to the right.
   This helps to build lateral movement, essential for boxing.

4. Boxer's Skip

Begin with a basic jump rope technique.

Shift your weight from one leg to the other.

Allow the non-weighted foot to kick slightly out to the side.

This helps to mimic the footwork found in boxing and can improve balance.

Strategies for Beginners:

Start Slow, don't worry about speed at first. Focus on finding a rhythm and maintaining consistent jumps. Add Variety, mix these exercises within your routine to keep it engaging and beneficial. Jump rope exercises can significantly contribute to a boxer's agility, footwork, stamina, and overall conditioning. For beginners, these exercises offer a foundation to build upon as skills improve.

4

Running

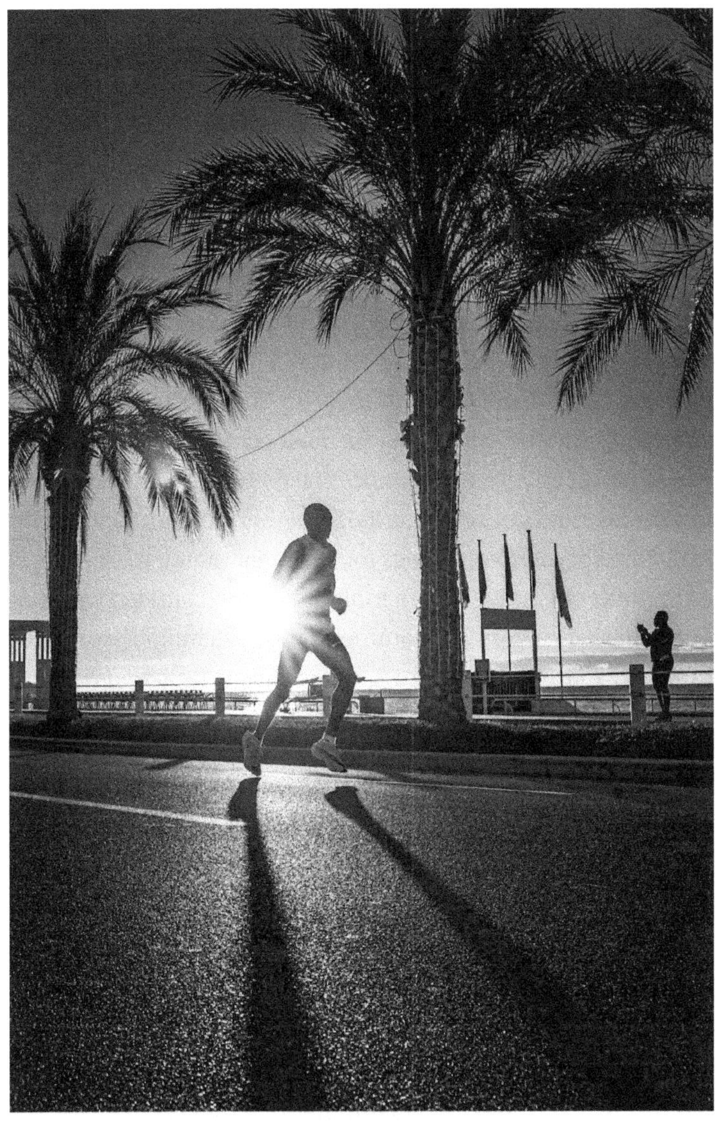

Running for Cardio Strength

Now that you are warmed up and have broken a sweat from jump roping, it is time to go for a run or a jog (depending on what pace of speed you feel is right for you). The purpose of running is to build leg strength as well as cardio endurance in your lungs. In my opinion, having high endurance is the most important prerequisite for boxing workouts. Without that, you just can't box for longer than a minute.

For this chapter, it is vital that you have comfortable sneakers that support your arches and ankles. There are many brands, and I've tried many of them myself. You just have to pick a sneaker brand that gives you the most comfort while allowing you to run at any pace you want. The point is to build strength in your legs and get better cardio. Whether it's short sprints for explosive speed or longer jogs for sustained stamina, running is a simple yet effective tool in molding a well-rounded workout enthusiast. I'm gonna recommend that you build three miles into your routine. Not all three miles have to be actual running or jogging - you can walk part of the way and mix running with walking throughout the workout.

Running Variations for Beginner Boxers

1. **Steady-State Running**

- **Objective:** To build a cardiovascular base and improve overall endurance.
- **Method:** Run at a consistent, moderate pace for a set distance or time (e.g., 30 minutes or 3 miles).
- **Frequency:** 2-3 times per week.

1. **Interval Running**

- **Objective:** To enhance speed and recovery time.
- **Method:** Alternate between periods of high-intensity running and low-intensity jogging or walking. For example, 1 minute of sprinting followed by 2 minutes of walking, repeated for 20-30 minutes.
- **Frequency:** 1-2 times per week.

1. **Hill Running**

- **Objective:** To build leg strength and explosive power.
- **Method:** Find a hill and run up it at a challenging pace, then walk or jog back down for recovery. Repeat several times.
- **Frequency:** Once a week.

1. **Fartlek Training**

- **Objective:** To improve speed, endurance, and adaptability.
- **Method:** A less structured form of interval training. Mix steady running with periods of faster running at irregular intervals. For example, sprint between certain landmarks like lampposts or trees during a steady run.
- **Frequency:** 1-2 times per week.

1. **Long Slow Distance (LSD) Runs**

- **Objective:** To enhance endurance and mental toughness.
- **Method:** Run a longer distance than your regular runs at a slow, manageable pace. Focus on maintaining a steady rhythm.

- **Frequency:** Once a week, preferably on a non-training day.

16

5

Shadowboxing

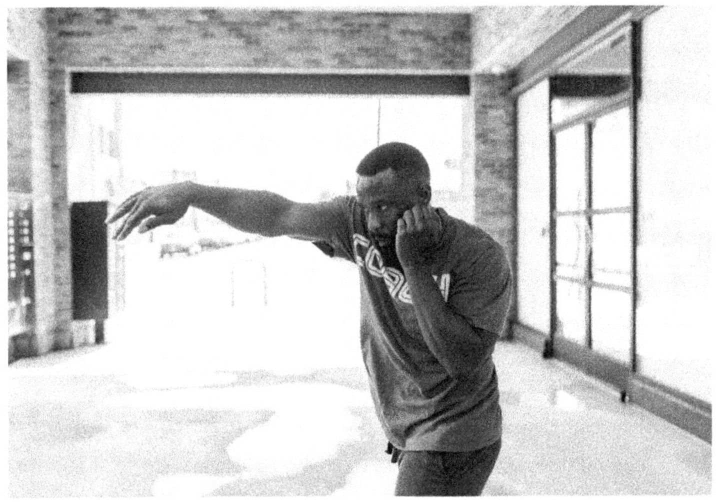

Visualize There's an Opponent in Front of You

The next step in your workout will be shadowboxing. Shadowboxing is a fundamental training technique in boxing, used by

beginners and professionals alike. It involves throwing punches at no particular target, allowing you to practice and refine your technique, footwork, and overall boxing strategy.

The Merits of Shadowboxing

1. **Technique Improvement:** Shadowboxing helps in refining your punching techniques and combinations without the need for a partner or equipment.
2. **Footwork and Movement:** It improves footwork, allowing you to practice moving around as you would in a real boxing match.
3. **Cardiovascular Fitness:** It's an excellent cardiovascular workout, enhancing your stamina and endurance.
4. **Mental Preparation:** It aids in mental training, helping you visualize opponents and plan strategies.
5. **Flexibility and Balance:** Regular shadowboxing increases flexibility and balance, crucial for boxing agility.

Shadowboxing Techniques

1. **Stance and Balance:** Begin in a proper boxing stance. Keep your feet shoulder-width apart, knees slightly bent, and your weight evenly distributed.
2. **Jab:** The jab is a quick, straight punch thrown with your lead hand. Extend your arm fully, rotating your fist to land with your knuckles.
3. **Cross:** The cross is a powerful straight punch thrown with your rear hand. Pivot your rear foot and rotate your hips as you punch, for added power.
4. **Hook:** The hook is a semi-circular punch thrown with either hand. Rotate your core and pivot your foot in the

direction of the punch.

5. **Uppercut:** The uppercut is an upward punch aimed at the opponent's chin. Drop your knees slightly and use your legs to generate power as you punch upward.

6. **Combination Punching:** Practice various combinations of these punches. Example: Jab-Cross-Hook.

7. **Footwork:** Incorporate movement with your punches. Move forward, backward, and side-to-side, maintaining your balance and stance.

Shadowboxing Exercises for Beginners

1. **Three-Minute Rounds:** Start with three-minute rounds of shadowboxing, focusing on different techniques. Gradually increase the number of rounds as your stamina improves.

2. **Mirror Training:** Stand in front of a mirror to observe and correct your form. Pay attention to your hand positioning and footwork.

3. **Visualization:** Imagine an opponent in front of you. This will help in strategizing your movements and punches.

4. **Speed Drills:** Focus on the speed of your punches in short bursts to improve your quickness.

5. **Endurance Training:** Incorporate longer rounds of shadowboxing to build endurance.

Conclusion

Shadowboxing is an invaluable tool in the arsenal of any aspiring boxer. It enhances technique, fitness, and mental preparation, forming the foundation of your boxing skills. Regular practice will lead to noticeable improvements in your boxing prowess, making it an essential component of your "Boxing Home Workouts for Beginners."

6

Stretching And Foam Rolling

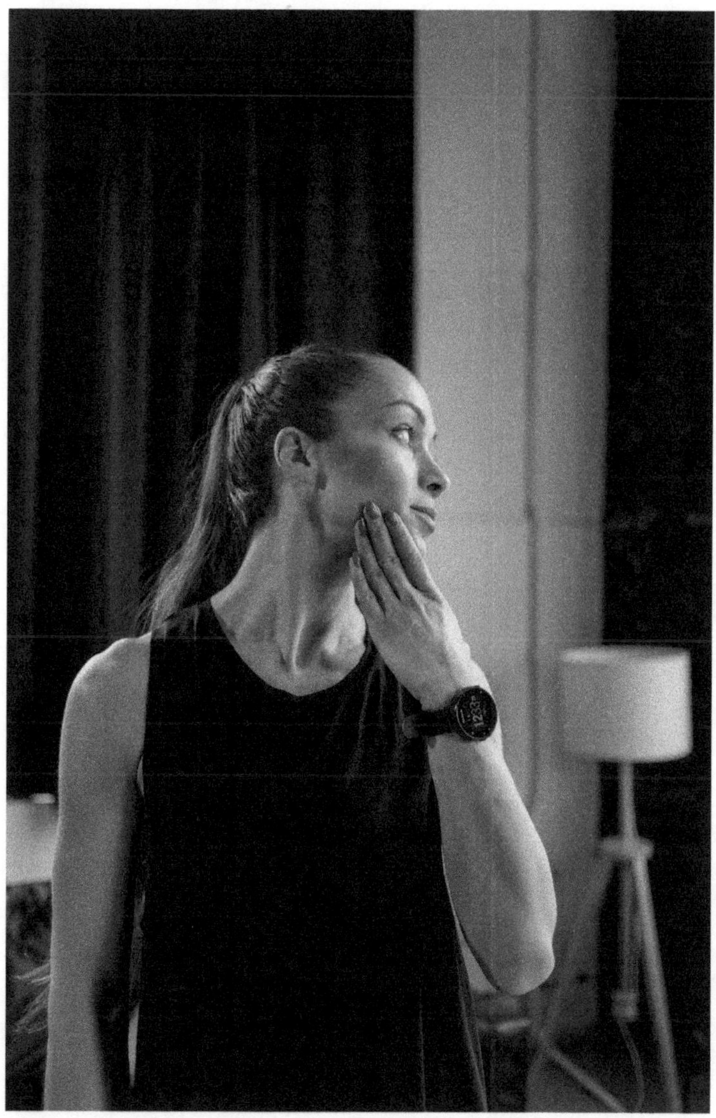

Keeping Yourself Loose and Stretched Out is Super Important for Boxing Workouts

Now that you are sweating and breathing deeply from running, it is time to stretch your warmed up muscles and tendons. Stretching is an essential part of any boxing workout, especially for beginners. It helps to increase flexibility, reduce the risk of injury, and improve overall performance. Here's a comprehensive guide for beginner stretching designed for a boxing workout:

Warm-up Stretches:

Perform these to prepare your muscles for more intense stretches. Do each stretch for about 10-15 seconds.

1. Neck Stretch

Gently tilt your head to one side, stretching the neck muscles. Hold and repeat on the other side.

2. Shoulder Circles

Rotate your shoulders forward and then backward in big circles.

3. Arm Swings

Swing your arms gently back and forth, above your head, to loosen the shoulder and chest muscles.

4. Hip Circles

Place your hands on your hips and make circles with your hips. Go both clockwise and counter-clockwise.

6. Leg Swings

Holding onto something for balance, swing one leg forward and backward.

Repeat with the other leg.

Intense Stretches:
These stretches should be held for 15-30 seconds to take stretching to the next level of your boxing workout.

7. Triceps Stretch
Reach one arm overhead, bending the elbow.
Gently push on the bent elbow with the opposite hand.
Repeat on the other side.

8. Shoulder Stretch
Bring one arm across your body.
Use the other arm to pull it closer to your chest.

9. Chest Stretch
Stand with feet shoulder-width apart.
Clasp hands behind back and gently pull arms upward.

10. Quadriceps Stretch
While standing, grab one ankle and pull it towards your glutes.
Keep knees together and hips straight.
Repeat on the other leg.

11. Hamstring Stretch
Sit with one leg extended and the other bent inward.
Reach toward the extended foot, feeling a stretch in the hamstring.

12. Calf Stretch
Step one foot back, pressing the heel into the floor.

Bend the front knee, feeling a stretch in the calf of the back leg.

13. Hip Flexor Stretch

Kneel on one knee with the other foot in front, forming a 90-degree angle with the front knee.

Push hips forward slightly to stretch the hip flexors.

14. Spinal Twist

Lying on your back, bring one knee across your body.

Keep shoulders on the ground and turn your head to the opposite side.

Remember to perform these stretches with smooth and controlled movements. Breathing deeply and consistently will help you get the most benefit. If any stretch feels painful or overly uncomfortable, ease back. These stretches target the key muscle groups used in boxing, helping beginners to prepare for and recover from their workouts effectively.

Resistance Band Stretches:

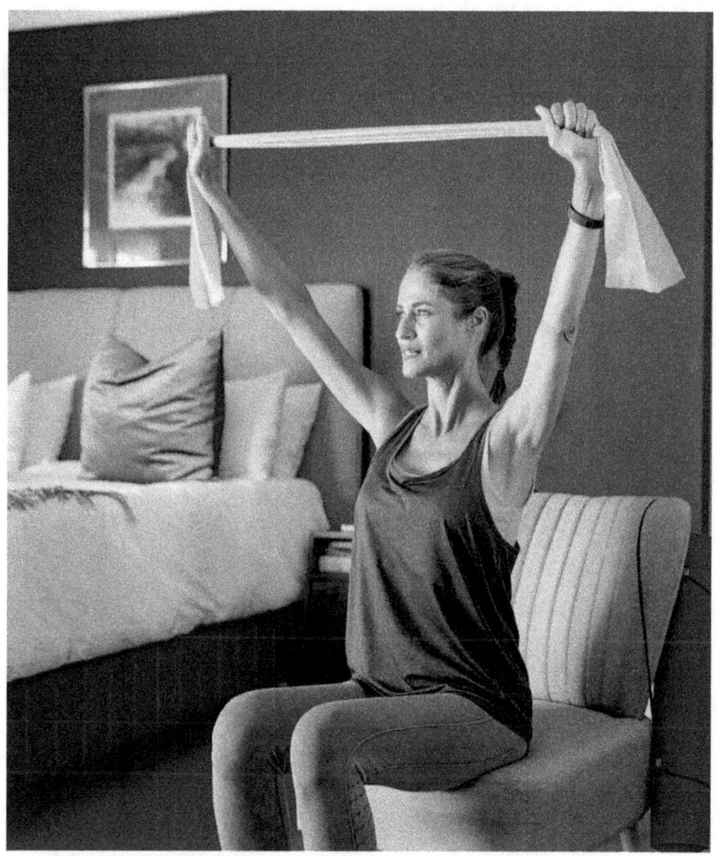

Stretching to increase your range of motion

As an addition to regular stretching, resistance bands offer a versatile way to loosen up those tight parts of your body. I prefer to use my resistance stretch band while sitting in a chair.

1. Shoulder Stretch

Sit upright in the chair.

Hold the band with both hands at shoulder-width apart.

Extend arms straight out in front and gently pull the band apart, feeling a stretch across the shoulders.

Hold and release slowly.

2. Tricep Stretch

Hold one end of the band above your head and the other end behind your back.

Gently pull the band, stretching the tricep of the arm overhead.

Switch sides and repeat.

3. Chest Stretch

Hold the band behind you with both hands, palms facing up.

Extend arms and gently pull the band apart to feel a stretch across the chest.

Hold and release.

4. Seated Leg Stretch

Sit at the edge of the chair.

Loop the band around the sole of one foot and hold both ends.

Extend the leg and gently pull the band towards you, stretching the hamstring.

Switch legs and repeat.

5. Ankle Stretch

Sit with feet flat on the floor.

Loop the band around one ankle.

Gently push the foot against the band's resistance, then pull it towards you.

Repeat with the other ankle.

4. Rotational Stretch

Hold the band with both hands, arms extended in front.
Rotate your upper body to one side, resisting with the band.
Return to center and repeat on the other side.

5. Upper Back Stretch

Hold the band with both hands wider than shoulder-width.
Extend arms overhead and gently pull the band apart, feeling
a stretch in the upper back.
Hold and release.

Tips for Chair Stretching with Resistance Bands:

- Maintain Proper Posture. Sit upright in the chair with feet
  flat on the floor. Keep your core engaged during stretches.
- Control Your Movements. Perform each stretch with slow
  and controlled movements to avoid unnecessary strain.
- Mind Your Breathing. Breathe deeply and consistently,
  exhaling as you stretch and inhaling as you return to the
  starting position.
- Using resistance bands for chair stretching is an effective
  way to increase flexibility, improve posture, and reduce
  muscle stiffness. These exercises can be easily incorporated
  into a daily workout routine, whether at home or the office,
  and tailored to individual needs and fitness levels.

Foam Rolling:

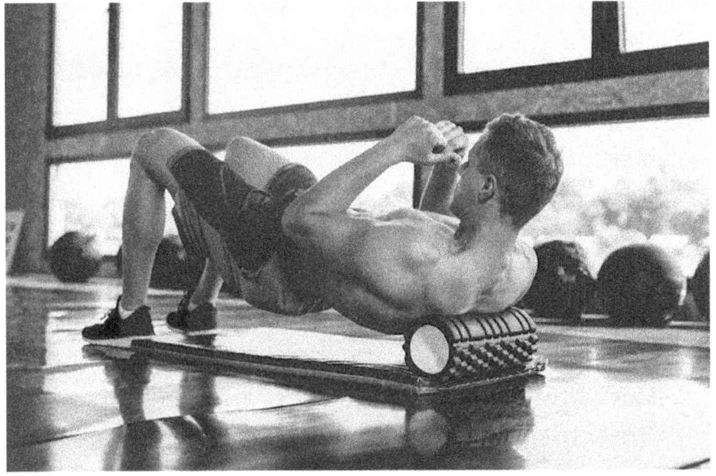

Foam rolling to reduce soreness and tightness

Also known as self-myofascial release, is an excellent tool for boxers at any level, including beginners. It helps in releasing muscle tightness, increasing blood flow, improving mobility, and aiding recovery. Here's a guide on how to use foam rolling effectively as part of a beginner's boxing workout routine:

1. Calves

Sit on the floor with legs extended.
Place the foam roller under one calf.
Lift your hips and roll back and forth over the calf muscle.
Repeat on the other leg.

2. Hamstrings

Place the foam roller under your thighs.

Support yourself with your hands behind you.

Roll back and forth from the knees to the glutes.

3. Quadriceps

Lie face down with the foam roller under your thighs.

Support your weight with your forearms and toes.

Roll from the hips to the knees, pausing at any tight spots.

4. Glutes

Sit on the foam roller with one ankle crossed over the opposite knee.

Lean slightly toward the side of the crossed leg.

Roll over the glute, focusing on any tight areas.

5. IT Band

Lie on your side with the foam roller under your hip.

Support yourself with your forearm and feet.

Roll down the side of your leg from hip to knee.

6. Upper Back

Lie on your back with the foam roller under your upper back.

Cross your arms over your chest or place hands behind your head.

Lift hips and roll from the upper to the mid-back.

7. Lats

Lie on your side with your arm extended and foam roller under the armpit area.

Roll up and down the side of your upper back.

Repeat on the other side.

Tips and Strategies for Beginners:

- Start Gentle. If you're new to foam rolling, begin with a softer foam roller and gradually increase pressure as you become more comfortable.
- Spend Time on Sore Spots. If you find a particular spot that's more sensitive or tight, spend some extra time there, gently rolling back and forth.
- Avoid Rolling Over Joints. Focus on the muscles and avoid rolling directly over joints or bones.
- Use Before and After Workouts. Foam rolling can be beneficial both pre and post-workout. Before workouts, it can help in warming up the muscles, and after workouts, it aids in recovery.
- Maintain Proper Form: Keep your core engaged, and maintain proper alignment to avoid unnecessary strain on other parts of your body.
- Hydrate: Drinking water post foam rolling can help in flushing out the toxins released during the rolling.

Foam rolling can be a powerful addition to a beginner's boxing routine. It aids in muscle recovery, flexibility, and overall performance, making it a valuable component for those starting out. Integrating these techniques can lead to a more effective and satisfying boxing workout experience.

7

Heavy Bag Work

These next workouts are foundational for building strength, explosiveness, and punching power. Whether your goal is to get your aggression and anger out on the bag or to build bigger muscles, the heavy bag is the right tool for that. But first let's make sure you have the proper equipment:

Heavy bag (should be half of your body weight), hanging in your garage from a ceiling beam. Or a standing heavy bag if you have nowhere to hang it and no garage.

Hanging Heavy Bag

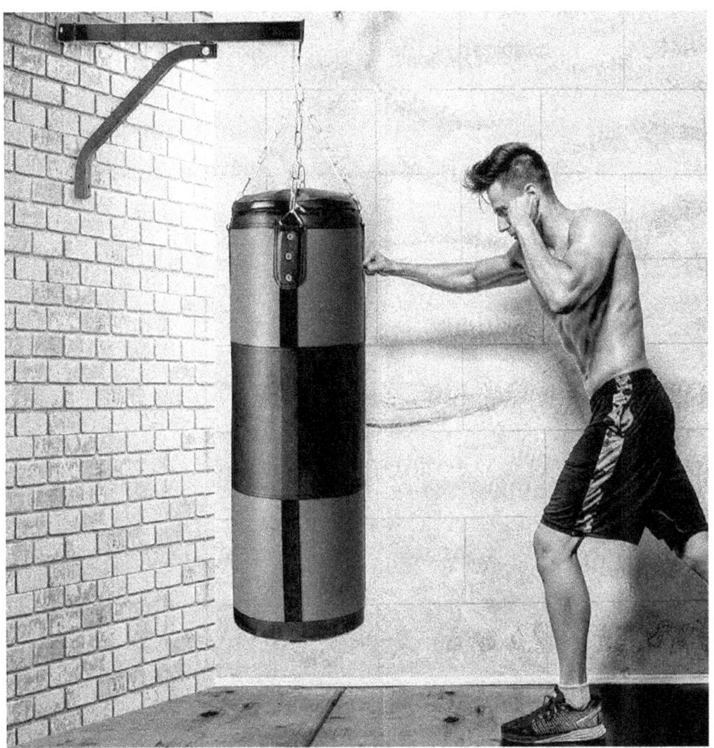

Description:

- A hanging heavy bag is typically suspended from the ceiling or a stand using chains or straps.
- It's often cylindrical and can vary in weight, commonly ranging from 40 to 150 pounds.

Advantages:

1. **Movement:** The bag swings when hit, offering a more

realistic simulation of an opponent's movement. This movement requires the boxer to adjust their footwork and timing for strikes.

2. **Feedback:** Provides better feedback upon impact, allowing for a more realistic experience in terms of how punches feel against an opponent.

3. **Versatility:** Suitable for a wider range of techniques, including punches, kicks, knees, and elbows, depending on its length.

Limitations:

1. **Space and Installation:** Requires a solid ceiling mount or a stand, which can take up significant space.

2. **Stability:** The ceiling or stand must be stable enough to support the bag's weight and movement, which might not be feasible in all training environments.

Standing Heavy Bag

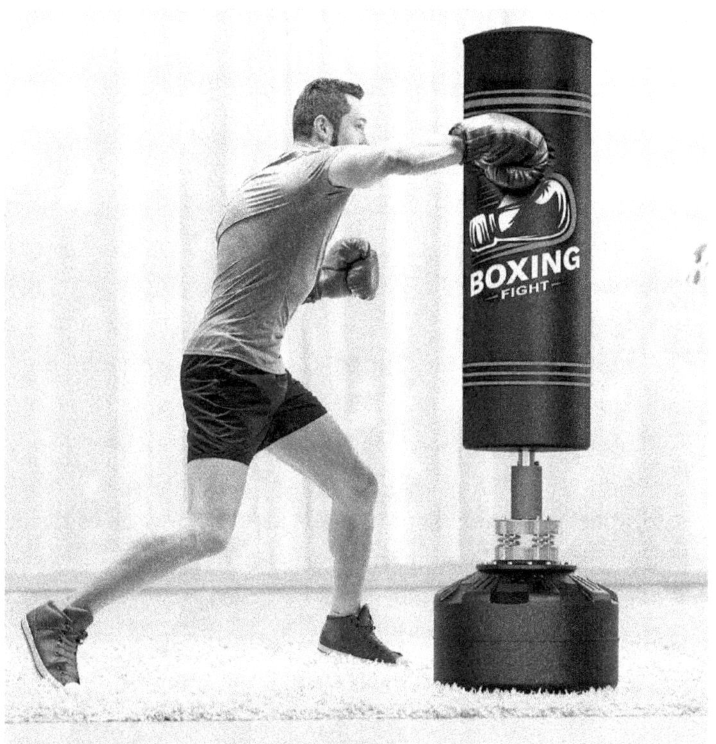

Description:

- A standing heavy bag stands upright on a base, which is often filled with water or sand to keep it stable.
- These bags can also vary in weight and size, and some models allow for height adjustments.

Advantages:

1. **Portability and Convenience:** Easier to move and set up, as

it doesn't require hanging. Ideal for home gyms or spaces where a hanging bag is not practical.

2. **Stability:** The base provides stability, and there's no risk of ceiling damage.
3. **Space-Saving:** Occupies less space and can be tucked away when not in use.

Limitations:

1. **Limited Movement:** The bag doesn't swing much, offering less realistic movement compared to a hanging bag. This can limit the development of advanced footwork and timing.
2. **Impact Feedback:** Some models may not provide as realistic feedback upon impact, especially for power punches or kicks.
3. **Base Obstruction:** The base can be an obstacle, especially for low kicks or movement around the bag.

The choice between a hanging heavy bag and a standing heavy bag depends on individual needs and training goals. If realism in movement and a wider range of techniques are priorities, and if space allows, a hanging heavy bag is preferable. For those with space constraints or who need a more portable and convenient option, a standing heavy bag is an excellent alternative. Both types offer effective workouts and can significantly benefit boxing training.

Boxing hand wraps, worn on your hands inside of gloves. Wraps are especially important for beginners, because as you start to punch with power, your unconditioned hands will need extra protection from getting cut and bruised. My favorite brand, due to their comfort, are TITLE Boxing Semi Elastic Hand Wraps. To learn how to wrap your hands properly, please refer to numerous YouTube tutorial videos online.

Boxing gloves, 16oz if you weigh over 150 lbs, or 10oz gloves if you weigh under 150 lbs.

Next, let's cover proper stance and the basic punches we'll be working with.

Boxing Stance

A good stance will keep you grounded and more confident to throw the necessary punches. The boxing stance is the foundation of a boxer's technique, providing stability, balance, and the ability to attack or defend effectively. Here's how to adopt the correct boxing stance for both orthodox (right-handed) and southpaw (left-handed) practitioners:

<u>Orthodox Stance (For Right-Handed Fighters)</u>

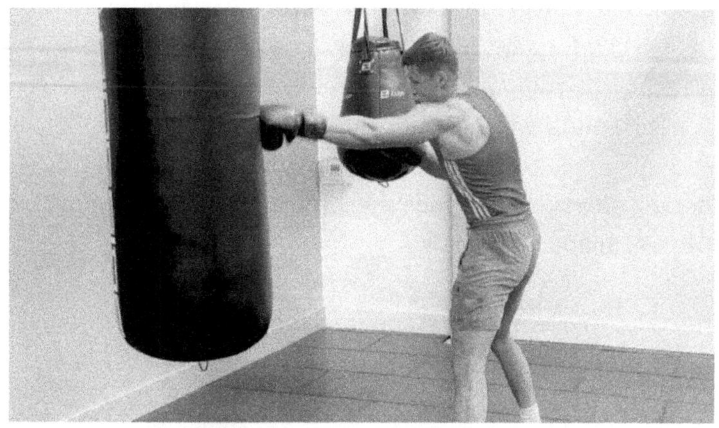

1. Feet Position

Stand with your feet shoulder-width apart. Place your left foot forward and your right foot back, keeping them aligned diagonally. Your back foot's heel may be slightly off the ground.

2. Knee Bend

Slightly bend your knees to enhance stability and mobility.

3. Hand Position

Keep your left fist at eye level and your right fist next to your chin. Your palms should face your face, and elbows should be tucked in close to the body to protect the ribs.

4. Chin and Head

Tuck your chin down into your chest, and keep your eyes on your bag. Your head should be behind your gloves.

5. Torso and Hips

Your upper body should be slightly turned to present a smaller target. Rotate your hips slightly to align with your back foot.

6. Weight Distribution

Balance your weight equally between both feet to ensure quick movement in any direction.

<u>Southpaw Stance (For Left-Handed Fighters)</u>

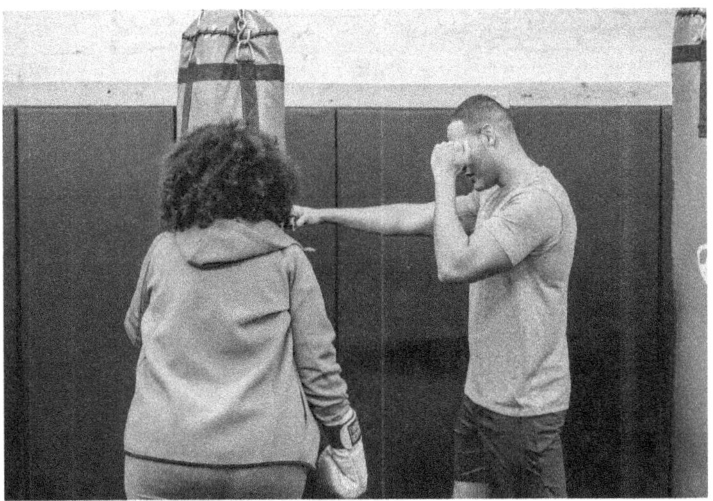

1. Feet Position

Similar to the orthodox stance but reversed. Your right foot is forward, and your left foot is back, with the feet aligned diagonally.

2. Knee Bend

Same as the orthodox stance, with a slight bend in the knees.

3. Hand Position

Right fist at eye level, left fist next to the chin, palms facing your face, and elbows close to the body.

4. Chin and Head

Tuck the chin, and keep eyes on the bag, with the head behind the gloves.

5. Torso and Hips

Turn your upper body slightly to the right and align your hips with the back foot.

6. Weight Distribution

Balance the weight equally between both feet.

Punches We'll be Working With

I. The Jab

Imagine a sword in a knight's hand - swift, precise, and the first line of attack. In boxing, the jab is that sword. Let's learn to wield it!

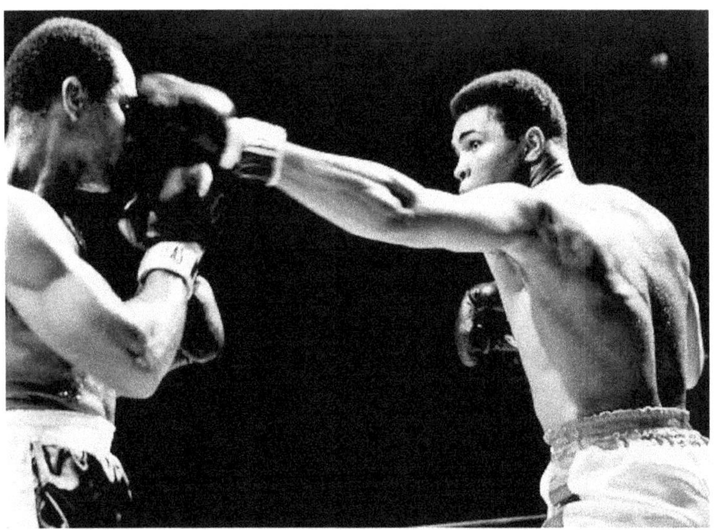

Anatomy of a Jab:

1. Lead Hand

The jab is thrown with the lead hand (left hand for orthodox fighters, right for southpaws).

2. Straight Line

The punch should travel in a straight line from the guard position to the target.

3. Rotation

Slight rotation of the forearm as the punch is thrown.

4. Recovery

Quick retraction back to guard position.

Workout routine: Three minute intervals, with 30 second

breaks. Repeat as many as you like. Jab the bag, just throw as many accurate and extended jabs as possible. You can throw at eye level, or to the body's stomach level if you bend your knees.

II. The Cross

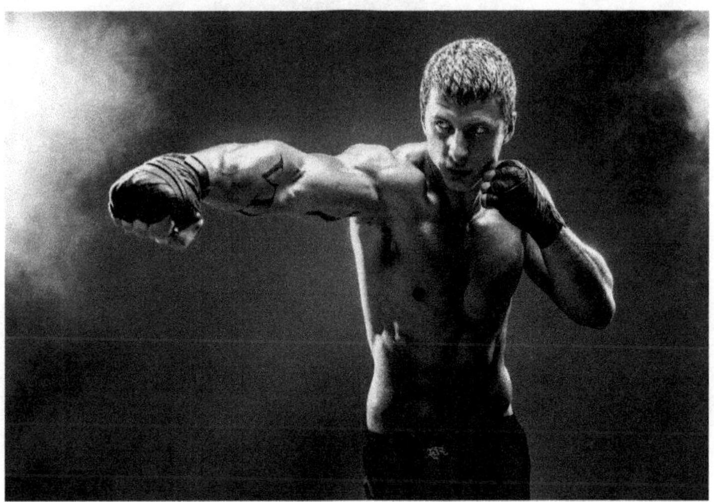

The cross, also known as a straight, is one of the fundamental punches in boxing. It's a powerful and direct strike typically thrown with the rear hand, allowing for a strong follow-through. For beginners, understanding and practicing the cross is vital to building a well-rounded skill set.

1. Stance and Positioning

Feet: Maintain a stable boxing stance with the rear foot

slightly behind.

Hands: Your front hand should be up, protecting your face, and your rear hand near your chin, ready to punch.

Body Alignment: Keep your body slightly angled, with your shoulders relaxed.

2. Executing the Cross

Pivot: As you begin to throw the punch, pivot on the ball of your rear foot, turning your hip and shoulder forward.

Extension: Extend your rear arm straight out, aiming for the target.

Wrist: Rotate your wrist so that the knuckles are horizontal at the point of impact.

Power: The power comes from the legs and hips, not just the arm. Feel the energy travel from the ground up.

3. Return and Defense

Recoil: After striking, quickly bring your hand back to the defensive position.

Balance: Maintain your balance to be ready for the next move or to defend against a counterpunch.

Workout routine: Three minute intervals, with 30 second breaks. Repeat as many as you like. Throw one jab followed by a cross, throw as many of these combos as possible. You can throw at eye level, or to the body's stomach level if you bend your knees. These are known as "one two" combos.

III. The Hook

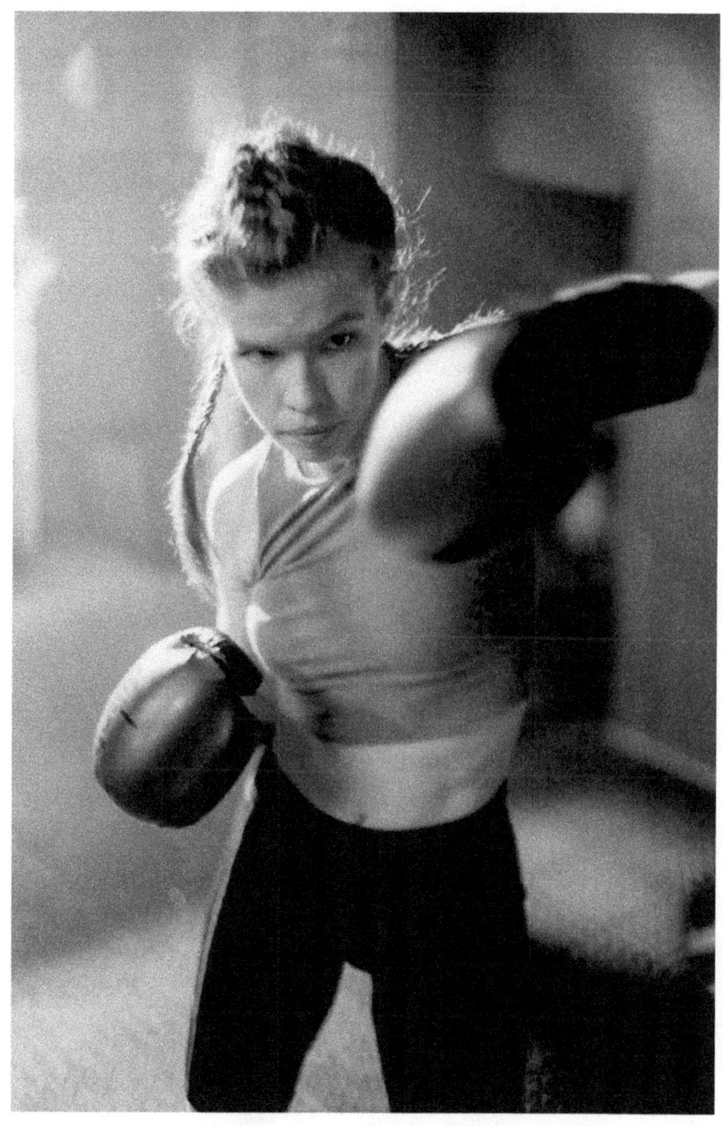

The boxing hook is a fundamental punch that's essential for anyone stepping into the world of boxing, even beginners. The hook is a powerful, semi-circular punch that comes from the side. It's one of the core punches in boxing and can be a fight-ending blow when executed properly. Unlike straight punches like the jab or cross, the hook travels in an arc, targeting the opponent's head or body.

Why Learn the Hook?

- Efficiency: The hook can be thrown quickly from a defensive position.
- Power: It utilizes the rotation of the hips and core, generating tremendous force.
- Versatility: It can target different areas, such as the head, jaw, or ribs, making it a strategic weapon.

How to Throw a Hook: A Step-by-Step Guide for Beginners

1. Starting Position
Stand in your boxing stance with your hands up, protecting your face.

2. Turn the Core
Begin the hook by rotating your core and hips, not just your arm. This is where the punch's power comes from.

3. Form the Hook
With a bent elbow, swing your arm in a horizontal arc towards the target. Your hips, and shoulders should swing in the same direction.

4. Aim with Precision

Focus on the heavy bag target, whether it's the opponent's head or body. The knuckles of your lead hand should connect with the target. Make the intention of 'punching through' the bag.

5. Protect Yourself

Keep your other hand up to protect your face, and don't overextend the punch; control is key.

6. Recover Quickly

Return to your starting position, ready for the next move.

Workout routine: Three minute intervals, with 30 second breaks. Repeat as many as you like. Throw one jab followed by a cross, followed by a lead hand hook to the head, followed by a rear hand hook to the body. These are known as "one two three" combos.

Common Mistakes to Avoid:

- Using Only the Arm. The power comes from the hips and core, not just swinging the arm.
- Dropping the Guard. Always keep the other hand up to defend against counterpunches.
- Overreaching. Overextending leaves you vulnerable. Practice control and precision.

IV. Uppercut

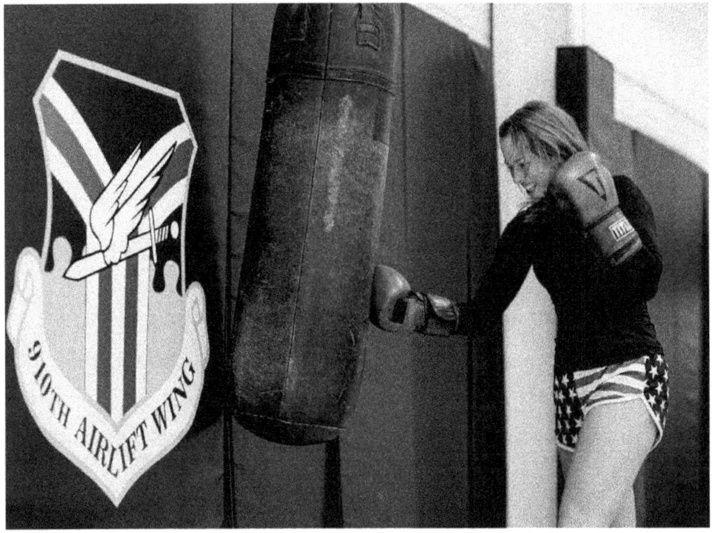

Practicing the Uppercut on the Heavy Bag

The uppercut is a potent punch in boxing, effective in breaking through an opponent's defense. Practicing on a heavy bag allows you to develop power, accuracy, and technique for this crucial punch.

Understanding the Heavy Bag for Uppercut Training

A heavy bag is a durable, weighted bag used for boxing training. It simulates the resistance and feel of an actual opponent, making it ideal for practicing punches like the uppercut.

Fundamentals of the Uppercut

1. **Stance:** Start in your boxing stance with your feet shoulder-width apart and knees slightly bent.
2. **Hand Positioning:** Keep your hands up, protecting your

face. The hand not throwing the uppercut should remain defensive.

3. **Execution:** The uppercut is thrown in an upward motion, targeting the opponent's chin or body. Use your legs and hips to generate power, pivoting slightly for added force.

Techniques for Practicing Uppercuts on a Heavy Bag

1. **Single Uppercuts:** Begin with single uppercuts to focus on form. Alternate between left and right hands, ensuring proper body movement and hand positioning.
2. **Uppercut Combinations:** Mix uppercuts with other punches (e.g., jab-uppercut-hook) to practice flowing movements.
3. **Close-Range Practice:** Stand closer to the bag to simulate the short range at which uppercuts are typically thrown.

Drills for Improving Uppercut Effectiveness

1. **Power Drills:** Throw consecutive uppercuts at full strength to build power. Focus on driving through with your legs and hips.
2. **Speed Drills:** Practice quick, successive uppercuts to increase speed and agility.
3. **Endurance Rounds:** Perform extended rounds focusing solely on uppercuts to build stamina and muscle endurance.

Tips for Safe and Effective Uppercut Practice

1. **Wrist Alignment:** Keep your wrist straight and aligned with your forearm to prevent injury.

2. **Breathing:** Exhale sharply with each punch to maintain rhythm and power.
3. **Focus on Form:** Prioritize proper technique over power to develop effective muscle memory.

Mastering the uppercut on a heavy bag is a vital step in developing your boxing skills. Regular practice focusing on power, speed, and technique will enhance your proficiency with this punch. As you progress, the uppercut will become a key component in your workouts, making your "Boxing Home Workouts for Beginners" more dynamic and effective.

8

Boxing Combo Drills on the Heavy Bag for Beginners

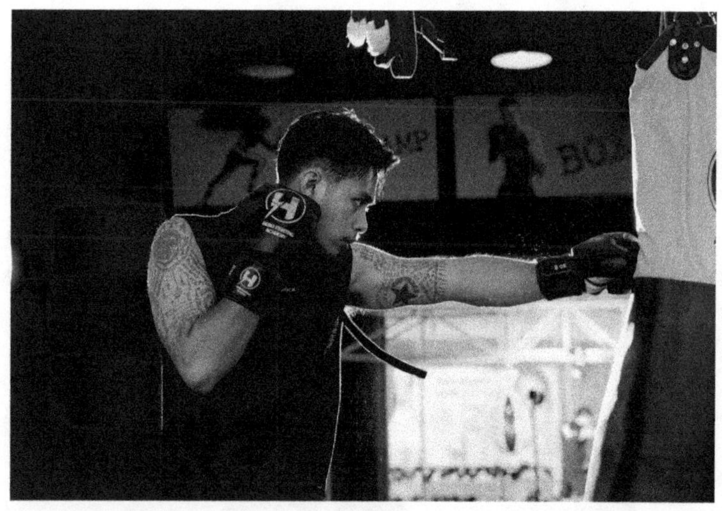

Practicing Combos of All The Various Punches Together

Combination punching is a fundamental skill in boxing, involving the rapid execution of a series of punches. Practicing combo drills on a heavy bag helps beginners develop rhythm, power, and fluidity in their punching sequences.

The Importance of Combo Drills

1. **Skill Integration:** Combo drills integrate various punches, helping you learn how to transition smoothly between them.
2. **Strategic Thinking:** They train you to think strategically about punch selection and sequencing.
3. **Rhythm and Timing:** These drills improve your rhythm and timing, essential for effective boxing.
4. **Endurance and Power:** They also enhance your endurance and power by simulating the intensity of a real boxing bout.

Fundamental Combos for Beginners

1. **Jab-Cross (1-2 Punch):** The most basic and essential combo. The jab (lead hand) is followed quickly by the cross (rear hand).
2. **Jab-Cross-Hook:** Add a hook (either hand) after the 1-2 punch for a three-punch combination.
3. **Cross-Hook-Cross:** This combo starts with the power punch (cross) followed by a hook and another cross.
4. **Jab-Uppercut-Cross:** A varied combination that includes an uppercut, introducing the concept of vertical punching.

Combo Drill Techniques on the Heavy Bag

1. **Start Slow:** Begin by throwing each combo slowly to understand the movement and flow of the punches.

2. **Gradually Increase Speed:** As you become comfortable, gradually increase the speed of your combos.
3. **Focus on Form:** Ensure each punch is executed with proper form before increasing speed or power.
4. **Use Full Range of Motion:** Extend your arms fully for jabs and crosses, and rotate your torso for hooks and uppercuts.

Drills for Practice

1. **Repetition Drills:** Repeat the same combo for a set number of rounds to build muscle memory.
2. **Varying Combos:** Alternate between different combos within a round to keep the training dynamic.
3. **Power Rounds:** Focus on throwing each combo with maximum power for short bursts.
4. **Endurance Rounds:** Practice combos at a consistent pace for longer rounds to build stamina.

Tips for Effective Combo Training

1. **Breathing:** Exhale sharply with each punch to maintain rhythm and avoid fatigue.
2. **Footwork:** Incorporate movement around the bag to simulate a real fight scenario.
3. **Visualize an Opponent:** Imagine responding to an opponent's movements and openings.
4. **Rest and Recovery:** Take adequate rest between rounds to maintain the quality of your training.

Combo drills on the heavy bag are essential for developing your boxing technique, power, and endurance. By regularly practicing these drills, you will enhance your ability to execute combinations fluidly and effectively, a crucial skill for any boxer. Remember, consistency is key in your "Boxing Home Workouts for Beginners," and these combo drills will serve as a solid foundation for your boxing journey.

Integrating Low and High Punches in Heavy Bag Combo Drills for Beginners

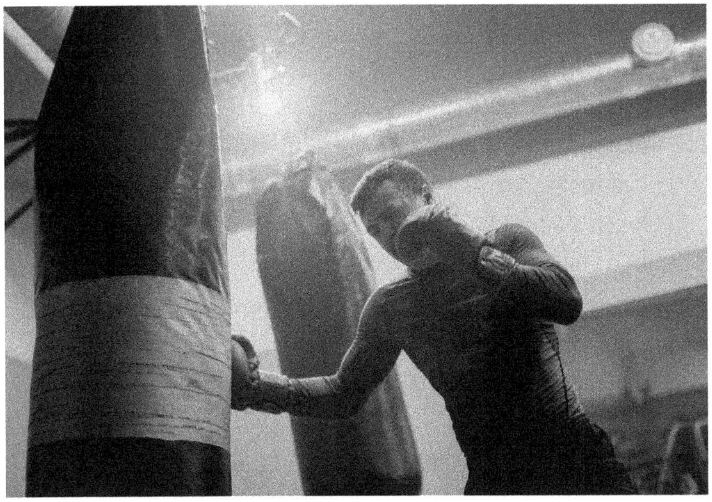

It's Time to Combine Low and High Punches

In boxing, varying the height of your punches in combinations (combos) can create a dynamic and unpredictable attack. Integrating low (body) and high (head) punches in your heavy bag drills can significantly enhance your boxing skills, teaching you how to target different areas effectively.

Understanding Low and High Punches

1. **High Punches:** These are aimed at the head of an opponent. Common high punches include jabs, crosses, hooks, and uppercuts aimed at the chin or sides of the head.
2. **Low Punches:** These target the body, particularly the abdomen and ribs. Low jabs, crosses, and especially hooks and uppercuts are effective here.

The Benefits of Mixing Low and High Punches

1. **Offensive Diversity:** Varying punch heights keeps your opponent guessing, making your offense less predictable.
2. **Defensive Strategy:** It forces your opponent to defend on multiple levels, potentially creating openings.
3. **Increased Power:** Proper body mechanics used in low punches can generate significant power.
4. **Stamina and Endurance:** This approach demands more from your body, enhancing your conditioning.

Integrating Low and High Punches in Combo Drills

1. **Start with Basic Combos:** Begin with simple combinations, like a high jab followed by a low cross, to get used to changing punch levels.
2. **Progress to Advanced Combos:** As you get comfortable, integrate more complex sequences, like a high jab-cross followed by a low hook, then finishing with a high uppercut.
3. **Emphasize Body Movement:** When throwing low punches,

it's essential to bend at the knees and waist, not just lower your arms.

4. **Maintain Guard:** Keep your guard up, especially when targeting the body, as your head becomes more exposed.

Sample Combo Drills with Low and High Punches

1. **Jab (High) - Cross (Low) - Hook (High):** This combo starts with a high jab, quickly followed by a low cross to the body, and finishes with a high hook.
2. **Double Jab (High) - Uppercut (Low) - Cross (High):** Begin with two high jabs, drop down for a low uppercut, then rise again for a high cross.
3. **Cross (High) - Hook (Low) - Hook (High):** Start with a high cross, then a low hook to the body, followed by another hook to the head.
4. **Uppercut (Low) - Uppercut (High) - Cross (High):** Deliver a low uppercut, followed by a high uppercut with the same hand, and finish with a high cross.

Tips for Effective Low and High Punch Training

1. **Focus on Form:** Ensure your low punches are executed with proper bending and pivoting.
2. **Controlled Movements:** Avoid overextending or dropping your guard when switching between low and high punches.
3. **Breathing Technique:** Maintain rhythmic breathing, exhaling with each punch.
4. **Visualization:** Imagine an opponent's body and head while switching between punch heights.

Incorporating both low and high punches in your heavy bag combo drills is an excellent way to enhance your boxing technique. This approach not only improves your offensive capabilities but also significantly boosts your defensive skills by preparing you to attack and defend on multiple levels. Regular practice of these varied combos will be a key part of your "Boxing Home Workouts for Beginners," making you a more versatile and formidable workout enthusiast.

9

Calisthenics

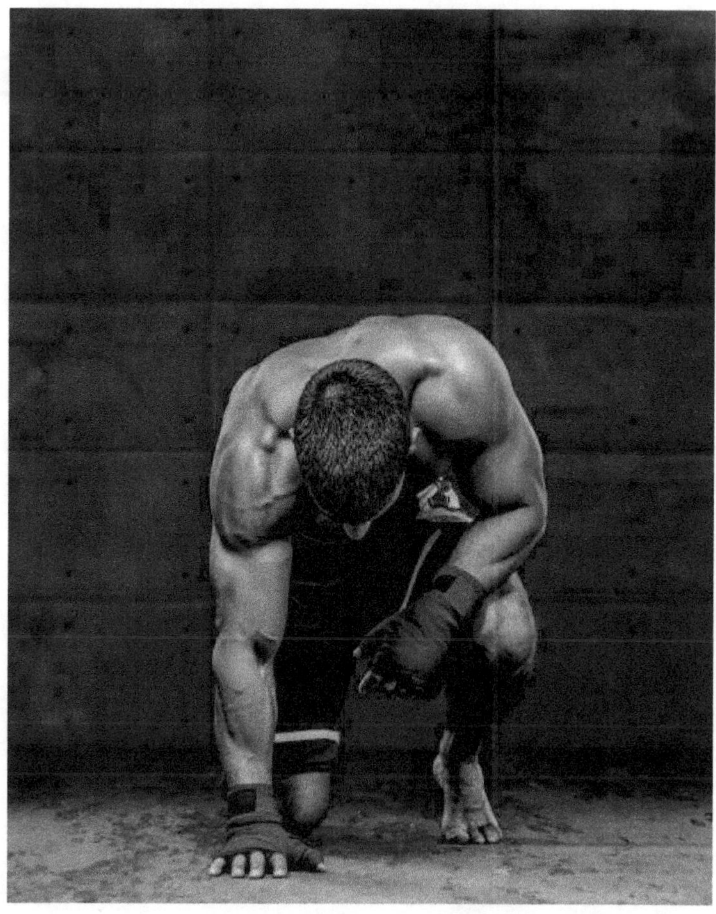

A boxing workout would not be complete without calisthenic exercises. At the end of each workout at the boxing studio, we do lots of calisthenics. These include push-ups, sit-ups and squats. This ensures that your muscles get toned and continue to become stronger for your next workout.

I. Push-Ups

I personally do all my push-ups on my knuckles, and preferably on a hard surface (i.e. garage). But feel free to adjust this to your environment.

1. There are two important elements in boxing push-ups - *breath* **and** *arm extension.*

I recommend inhaling on the down movement, and exhaling on the up movement. Feel free to change this up as you feel comfortable.

2. Train to breathe under stress.

Breathing keeps more oxygen pumping into your muscles.

3. Make sure you fully extend your arm each time you come up in a push-up.

This simulates real punches and their motion.

Workout routine: You can start out with as many push-ups as you can handle in the beginning. Build up from there and stay consistent, and you'll be doing dozens of them after several months.

II. Sit-Ups

Sit-ups are a critical component of boxing training as they help strengthen the core muscles, vital for stability, power, and endurance in the ring. Here's a sit-ups workout tailored for boxing beginners, designed to be both challenging and achievable:

1. Traditional Sit-ups

Position: Lie on your back, knees bent, feet flat, and hands behind your head.

Action: Engage the core to lift your upper body toward your knees.

Reps: 3 sets of 12.

Rest: 30 seconds between sets.

2. Leg Raise Sit-ups

Position: Lie down, legs extended, hands behind your head.

Action: As you sit up, lift one leg, aiming to touch your opposite elbow.

Reps: 2 sets of 10 for each leg.

Rest: 30 seconds between sets.

3. Plank to Sit-up Transition

Position: Start in a plank position.

Action: Transition to a seated position and perform a sit-up, then return to the plank.

Reps: 2 sets of 8.

Rest: 45 seconds between sets.

4. Russian Twists with Sit-up

Position: Sit with knees bent, lean back slightly.

Action: Perform a Russian twist, then lower into a sit-up position and sit back up.

Reps: 2 sets of 10.

Rest: 30 seconds between sets.

5. Weighted Sit-ups (Optional and only if comfortable)

Position: Same as traditional sit-ups but holding a light weight plate or dumbbell.

Action: Perform sit-ups as usual.
Reps: 2 sets of 10.
Rest: 30 seconds between sets.
Cool Down

6. Stretching

Finish with a gentle cobra pose stretching focusing on the core and breathing deeply to aid recovery.

Workout routine: You can start out with as many sit-ups as you can handle in the beginning. Build up from there and stay consistent, and you'll be able to do hundreds of them after several months.

III. Squats

Legs are the pillars of a boxer. Strong legs mean powerful punches, rapid movements, and enduring rounds. It all begins with the humble squat. Squats are a fundamental exercise for strengthening the legs, core, and back muscles, and improving overall power and balance. Here's a beginner-friendly squat routine specifically designed for aspiring boxers:

1. Stance and Posture

Feet shoulder-width apart
Toes slightly turned out
Chest up, shoulders back
Core engaged

2. Execution

Slowly lower down, pushing hips back
Keep knees in line with toes

Maintain a straight back
Aim for thighs parallel to the ground
Repeat 3 sets of 10 reps

3. Safety and Tips
Keep weight on the heels
Avoid letting knees go past toes
Breathe in on the way down, exhale on the way up
Consider using a mirror for form checks

Workout routine: You can start out with as many squats as you can handle in the beginning. Just build up from there and stay consistent, and you'll be doing dozens of them after several months.

10

Systema Pushups - Enhancing Boxing Performance

Systema, a Russian martial art, offers unique training exercises, including Systema pushups, known for their holistic approach to improving strength, flexibility, and mental endurance. These pushups are particularly beneficial for boxers, aiding in the development of core strength, shoulder stability, and overall physical conditioning.

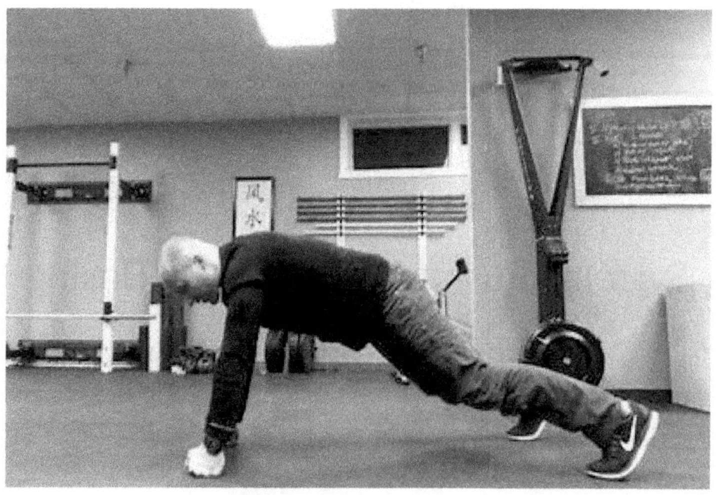

Understanding Systema Pushups

Systema pushups differ from traditional pushups in their emphasis on fluid, continuous motion and the integration of breathing techniques. They focus on full-body engagement and often incorporate varying hand positions and movement patterns.

Benefits of Systema Pushups for Boxers

1. **Enhanced Core Strength:** These pushups engage the core muscles more intensely than standard pushups, providing better stability and power for punches.
2. **Shoulder Stability and Flexibility:** The varied hand positions and movements strengthen and mobilize shoulder joints, vital for boxing.
3. **Improved Mental Focus:** The integration of breathing and

movement enhances mental focus and endurance.

4. **Greater Body Awareness:** Systema pushups encourage a deeper awareness of body mechanics and alignment.

Introduction to Specific Systema Pushups

Systema pushups are designed to enhance strength, flexibility, and mental focus. For beginner boxers, mastering these pushups can lead to significant improvements in boxing performance. Below are detailed instructions for specific Systema pushup variations tailored for beginners.

1. Standard Systema Pushup

Objective: To develop controlled, full-body strength and enhance breathing coordination.

Instructions:

1. **Starting Position:** Begin in a standard pushup position, with hands shoulder-width apart and feet together.
2. **Movement:** Slowly lower your body to the ground while inhaling deeply. Keep your body straight and core engaged.
3. **Breathing:** As you descend, breathe in deeply through the nose, filling your lungs completely.
4. **Push Up:** Exhale through the mouth as you push back up to the starting position.
5. **Pace:** The movement should be slow and controlled, focusing on the synchronization of breath with movement.

2. Knuckle Pushups

Objective: To strengthen the wrists and forearms, replicating the position of a boxing punch.

Instructions:

1. **Starting Position:** Make fists with both hands and set them on the ground in line with your shoulders, knuckles facing down.
2. **Movement:** Perform a pushup, maintaining balance on your knuckles.
3. **Wrist Alignment:** Ensure your wrists are straight and strong to avoid strain.
4. **Breathing:** Inhale on the way down and exhale on the way up, as with the standard pushup.

3. Wide Grip Pushups

Objective: To target the chest and shoulders more intensely.

Instructions:

1. **Starting Position:** Place your hands wider than shoulder-width apart, fingers pointing forward.
2. **Movement:** Lower your body until your chest is close to the ground, then push back up.
3. **Elbow Movement:** Your elbows should move out to the sides during the exercise.
4. **Breathing:** Maintain the same breathing pattern as in the standard pushup.

4. Single-Leg Pushups

Objective: To engage the core muscles and improve balance.

Instructions:

1. **Starting Position:** Begin in a standard pushup position, then lift one leg off the ground, keeping it straight.
2. **Movement:** Perform the pushup while maintaining the raised leg position.

3. **Balance:** Focus on keeping your body stable. Avoid tilting to one side.
4. **Breathing:** Follow the same breathing technique as in other variations.

General Tips for Beginners

- **Quality Over Quantity:** Focus on performing each pushup with proper form rather than on the number of pushups.
- **Progress at Your Own Pace:** Start with fewer repetitions and gradually increase as your strength improves.
- **Listen to Your Body:** If you feel any pain, especially in the wrists or shoulders, adjust your form or take a break.
- **Consistent Practice:** Regular practice is key to improvement. Aim to incorporate these pushups into your routine several times a week.
- **Focus on Form:** Maintain proper form to maximize benefits and prevent injury.
- **Mind-Muscle Connection:** Concentrate on the muscles being worked to enhance engagement and effectiveness.
- **Regular Variation:** Regularly change your pushup variations to challenge different muscle groups and avoid plateaus.
- **Focus on Breathing:** Inhale deeply as you lower your body and exhale as you push up.

For beginner boxers, Systema pushups offer a comprehensive way to build the strength, flexibility, and mental discipline needed in boxing. By starting with these foundational pushup variations and gradually increasing the complexity and intensity of your workouts, you'll build a solid base for more advanced boxing techniques. Remember, consistent practice and attention to form and breathing are essential for reaping the full benefits of these exercises in your "Boxing Home Workouts for Beginners."

11

Essential Recovery Techniques for Beginner Boxers

Recovery is a crucial component of any boxing training regimen, especially for beginners. It allows your body to heal and strengthen, reducing the risk of injury and improving overall performance.

Understanding the Need for Recovery

1. **Muscle Repair:** Boxing is physically demanding, causing micro-tears in the muscles that need time to heal.
2. **Prevent Overtraining:** Rest prevents overtraining syndrome, characterized by fatigue, decreased performance, and increased risk of injury.
3. **Mental Refreshment:** Recovery also gives you a mental break, which is essential for maintaining motivation and focus.

Core Recovery Strategies for Beginner Boxers

1. **Adequate Sleep:** Aim for 7-9 hours of quality sleep per

night to facilitate physical and mental recovery.

2. **Proper Nutrition:** Consume a balanced diet rich in proteins, carbohydrates, and healthy fats to aid muscle repair and energy replenishment.

3. **Hydration:** Stay well-hydrated to support overall health and optimal bodily functions.

Active Recovery Techniques

1. **Light Exercise:** Engage in light activities like walking, swimming, or yoga on rest days to promote blood circulation and muscle recovery.

2. **Stretching:** Regular stretching helps maintain flexibility, reduce muscle tightness, and prevent injuries.

3. **Foam Rolling:** Use a foam roller to perform self-myofascial release, aiding in muscle relaxation and recovery.

Passive Recovery Methods

1. **Rest Days:** Take complete rest days with no strenuous physical activity to allow your body to fully recover.

2. **Cold and Heat Therapy:** Use ice packs for acute injuries or soreness, and warm baths or heat packs to relax muscles and improve blood flow.

3. **Massage Therapy:** Consider professional massage therapy to reduce muscle stiffness and promote relaxation.

Post-Training Recovery Routine

1. **Cool Down:** After training, perform a cool-down routine

with light aerobic activity and stretching to gradually lower heart rate and relax muscles.

2. **Post-Workout Nutrition:** Consume a mix of protein and carbohydrates within 30 minutes of training to aid in muscle recovery and energy replenishment.
3. **Monitor Soreness and Fatigue:** Keep track of how your body feels. Persistent soreness or fatigue may indicate inadequate recovery.

Mental Recovery Techniques

1. **Mindfulness and Meditation:** Practice mindfulness or meditation to reduce stress and improve mental resilience.
2. **Adequate Leisure Time:** Ensure you have leisure time to relax and enjoy activities outside of boxing.

Recovery is as important as training in boxing. For beginners, it's crucial to incorporate various recovery techniques into your routine to ensure your body and mind are well-rested and ready for the next training session. By prioritizing recovery, you'll improve your performance, reduce the risk of injury, and enjoy a more sustainable and enjoyable boxing journey as part of your "Boxing Home Workouts for Beginners."

Final Words on Recovery

Common sense is always my advice for recovery. Drink plenty of water during your workouts. I drink three bottles of water, plus green tea throughout the day. Get a good night's sleep. Eat wholesome foods and lots of veggies for energy and improved blood flow.

12

Conclusion

Victory is Yours: A New Chapter in Your Fitness Journey

If you've made it this far, congratulations! You've successfully navigated the maze of boxing basics, techniques, and workout plans. Not only have you acquired a unique skill set, but you've also embarked on a transformative journey toward ultimate fitness and well-being. As we wrap up this guide, it's time to take a moment and appreciate the sweat, the commitment, and the willpower you've invested in yourself.

You stepped into this experience as a beginner, but you're walking away as someone far stronger, more disciplined, and most importantly, empowered. And while boxing is the medium we chose, the underlying triumph here is your renewed commitment to health and well-being.

Keeping the Game Alive

Now you have everything you need to achieve your fitness goals with boxing workouts for beginners, it's time to pass on your newfound knowledge and show other readers where they can find the same help.

Simply by leaving your honest opinion of this book on Amazon, you'll show other workout beginners where they can find the information they're looking for, and pass their passion for boxing home workouts forward.

Simply scan the QR code below to leave your review on Amazon:

QR code to leave your book review